30 DAYS
DIET DEVOTIONALS

Charlene M. Parrish, ND

I am a registered Doctor of Naturopathy and not a licensed Medical Doctor. Therefore, I do not practice "the application of scientific principles to prevent, diagnose, and treat physical and mental diseases, disorders, and conditions to safeguard the life and health of any woman and infant through pregnancy and parturition." I am an educator.

Charlene M. Parrish, ND
Doctor of Natural Health

About the Author

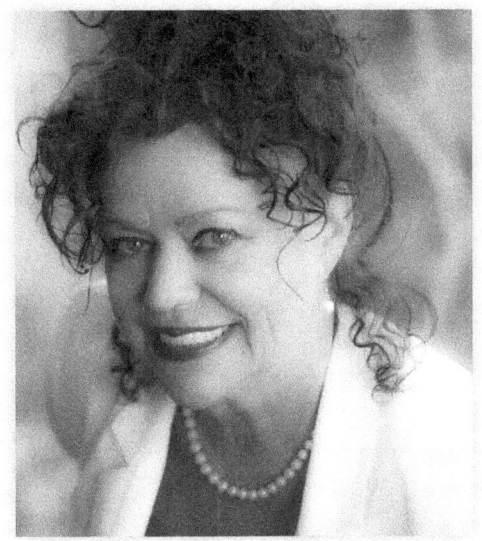

Charlene M. Parrish, ND holds a doctorate in naturopathic medicine and has over thirty years of natural health research. She is an international sought after teacher, writer and healer.

www.charleneparrish.com
www.30poundsin3weeks.com

Post Office Box 2122
Thomasville, GA 31799-2122
Charlene M. Parrish, ND

About the Author

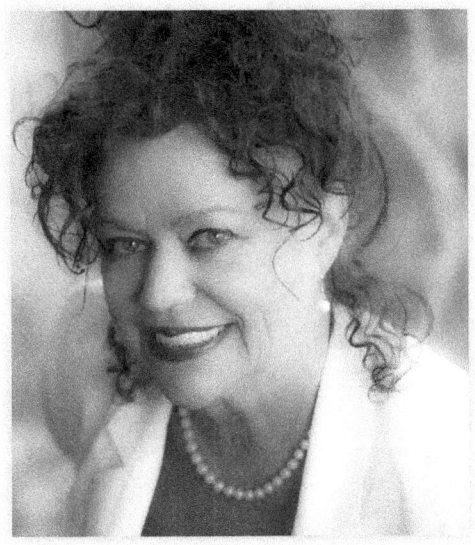

Charlene M. Parrish, ND holds a doctorate in naturopathic medicine and has over thirty years of natural health research. She is an international sought after teacher, writer and healer.

www.charleneparrish.com
www.30poundsin3weeks.com

Post Office Box 2122
Thomasville, GA 31799-2122
Charlene M. Parrish, ND

Table of Contents

A special thank you from my heart to Jim Spangler of worldaxisgroup@gmail.com for his inspired creative input into this book cover, and my life.

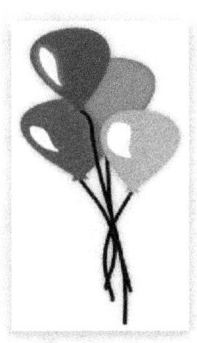

This book would not have been possible without the keen eye and tender heart of Alisha Wiggins who labored many hours over my ramblings, without even complaining. I pray Daddy multiply her precious time with her son back to her.

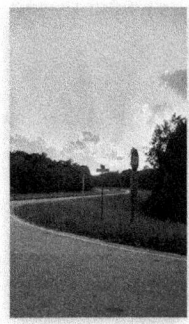

Foreword

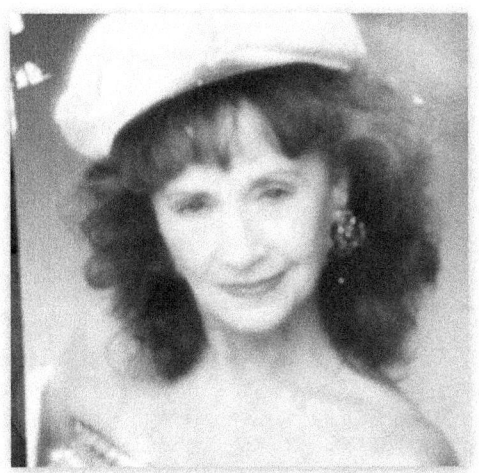

This book is dedicated to my Maudi, the great majorette of the Thomasville Marching Band who has told me every day of my life how beautiful I am. Mother believes you tell a child who they will be. She surrounded our world with scripture and even posted above the kitchen sink: "Whatsoever ye do, do it heartily as unto the Lord." These writings are my best attempt at just that.

Day One

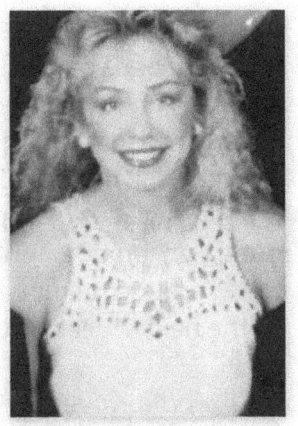

"Where there is no vision, the people perish." (Proverbs 29:18 KJV)

T oday is the first day of my diet and considered a "Load Day". In my book <u>30 Pounds in 3 Weeks</u>, I call these next couple of days of excessive eating "Love Days". You eat everything you think you might want for the next 3 weeks, especially high fat foods. Personally, I never eat sugar and limit my carbohydrates because these are my "trigger" foods to eat too much, but these load days are important.

You know how you feel at the end of Thanksgiving Day, especially that night after left-overs? You mutter things about never eating again.

Well, Load Days are like that. There are physical reasons, but most important are the spiritual and psychological parts. It is the beginning of the diet and you are preparing for the next few weeks.

One of my first steps to succeeding in this diet is preparation. I HAVE to rally some prayer partners now. The Word says, *"Without counsel plans fail, but with many advisors they succeed."* (Proverbs 15:22 ESV) People who really love me need to support this project I am starting. They need to understand it is not just a diet, but a very important commitment to my physical, mental and spiritual health. I need them to commit to pray for my daily focus and my success. Not everyone will understand. As a matter of fact, most of those around me will not. So it is important I choose my supporting friends with forethought.

I have to plan well. My vision needs to be clear to me, and to those I expect to support my diet journey. In my first book about my diet, I tell a humorous story about riding my bicycle wearing a big orange hunting vest with all my curls tucked under a black helmet. People were pointing and laughing, but after my 100 pound weight loss, people were rolling down their car windows and shouting encouragements and gesturing "thumbs ups". Those are the guys I need around me now. Those are the encouragers I need shouting at me for the next 3 weeks. I cannot do this on my own.

Karen has been my best friend for over forty years. We were single again together raising three small children, and that will surely help you grow up. She has always loved me just the way I am. Even if she's not happy with some decisions I have made, she has a way of encouraging me to do better the next time. She was a model and I always wanted to look like her; she admitted always wishing she had just said what I said. It is funny our differences seem to fade as we age. Karen has probably never seriously dieted in her life, but she will remember to pray for me and be a great encourager on this journey.

"Dear Father, please help me with these next few weeks of dieting. Thank you for the way you had me look at it like a fast; but, oh yeah I get to eat! Please help me focus on you and the prize at the end of this diet. I need you to be successful."

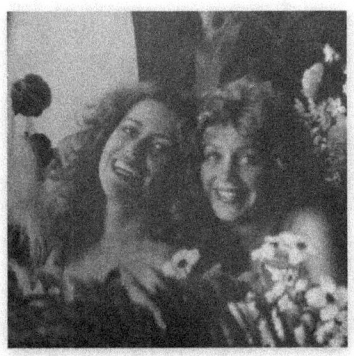

Who will you get to encourage you?

_____

_____

_____

_____

_____

_____

_____

_____

_____

_____

_____

_____

_____

_____

_____

Day Two

"*This is the day the Lord has made. Let us rejoice and be happy today!*" (Psalms 118:24 ERV)

Now you would think that would not be difficult today because it is another "Load Day", or "Love Day", but for some crazy reason I can stress out today just ANTICIPATING the next three weeks. But isn't today all I really have? Why in the world would I want to ruin a perfectly wonderful today of eating and drinking by worrying about tomorrow's dieting? My Daddy has this.

He said, "*Do not worry about your life, what you will eat or drink… Look at the birds of the air; they do not sow or reap…yet your heavenly Father feeds them. Are you not much more valuable…?*" (Mathew 6:25-26 NIV).

I will plan for my diet, but not worry. Today is a very precious day and I really am choosing to have a big celebration of who I am, and the fact that my Daddy has this.

How will you spend this day?

_____

_____

_____

_____

_____

_____

_____

_____

_____

_____

_____

_____

_____

_____

_____

_____

_____

_____

_____

_____

Day Three

"Therefore, take up the full armor of God, so that you will be able to resist in the evil day, and having done everything, to stand firm. Stand firm therefore, having girded your loins with truth, and having put on the breastplate of righteousness, and having shod your feet with the preparation of the gospel of peace; in addition to all, taking up the shield of faith with which you will be able to extinguish all the flaming arrows of the evil one. And take the helmet of salvation, and the sword of the Spirit, which is the word of God. With all prayer and petition pray at all times in the Spirit, and with this in view, be on the alert with all perseverance and petition for the saints, ..." (Ephesians 6: 13-18 NASB)

Somewhere along the way I figured out how important it is for me to put on my armor. We do start at the top of the head with the helmet as to remember it all, but my precious husband, David, and I pray this together every morning. It seems appropriate to start this new round of my diet totally armed with something stronger than my will power. Armed with just my will has never worked for me.

The scriptures that are right above these speak about being strong in the Lord and in the strength of his might, for our battles are not against flesh and blood, but rather against spiritual enemies. I believe this because I have been on a diet since third grade. Sometimes as a child I would just not eat or drink anything; yet, gain weight. If this were all a physical issue, wouldn't someone have cracked the code by now?

All the doctors want to talk about the physical, and there is some validity to not eating junk and monitoring what fuel you put in your engine. All the counselors want you to address your horrid past and I have seen major healings with my close girlfriend Robin's trapped emotion code work. All the preachers want you to just know Jesus. Have you ever been around someone so messed up that they were just incapable of even understanding anything about God? I personally believe we are all of that: body, mind and spirit. I have also seen some very smart people just not get some part of this and fail just as I have in the past. Why is it so different for me now? I have some ideas.

For sure, I do think differently now. I believe God really wants me to be healthy and prosperous; maybe not skinny, but a healthy weight. I believe God wants me to succeed in what makes me happy and that maybe my role is to make sure I seek only his perfect will for me just for today. If I really believe he really loves me, wouldn't I be able to trust even the asking him part? He doesn't want me to strive to figure it all out, but he wants me to be a little child and ask him.

One time I was envisioning myself praying at the feet of Jesus at what looked a lot like the huge statue of Abraham Lincoln. Right in the middle of my prayer, it was like God reached down and asked why I was way down there. He lifted me up to his breast and I blinked. That is so different than all my thoughts before.

So I put on my armor every morning, just in case. Maybe I do it just because he said to. David often adds, "And thank you, Lord, that my wife's belt of truth gets smaller every day."

"Dear Father, thank you that you just didn't leave me here to try and figure it all out by myself. I especially need your help for these next few weeks. Sometimes I do not make the best decisions so I ask you to help me. I want to stay close to you."

This diet is like a fast; but, oh yeah, I get to eat. Wouldn't I be crazy not to ask for help?

_____

_____

_____

_____

_____

_____

_____

_____

_____

_____

_____

_____

_____

_____

_____

_____

_____

_____

_____

Day Four

"Delight thyself in the Lord; and he shall give thee the desires of thine heart. Commit thy way unto the Lord; trust also in him; and he shall bring it to pass." (Psalms 37: 4-5 KJV).

have always heard the first part of that scripture, but only recently noticed the second verse. This understanding kind of changes things for me. Cheering because I am going to get the desires of my heart is one thing, but committing, trusting and waiting on God is a whole different deal. Everything about our present society seems to reward us for determined hard work. This diet is so odd because you don't get to set your "goals". You follow the rules, pray, and trust the Lord to bring it to pass. I learned it the hard way on my second round.

I had already started writing my book, <u>30 Pounds in 3 Weeks,</u> so of course I set my goal for another 30 pound weight loss. I stayed on the diet for 40 days and could only lose 29 and ½ pounds! If I had stayed on the diet for another month, I don't think I would have lost an ounce more. My Daddy seems to care way more about my relationship with him, than my diet. Don't get me wrong, I know how he wants me to be the best he made me to be. That includes my weight (his temple); but, he appears to be more interested in my spiritual growth along the way.

So yesterday was my first day of the Very Low Calorie Diet and today I am down 4 pounds. Isn't that crazy? Today I am praying to follow the rules and trust him to bring it to pass, but I will not be setting any weight loss goals. My goal will be to trust that he knows what is best, and his timing is perfect. God is so good.

What are your goals for these next few days? Do you think you can trust the one who made your beautiful body?

_____

_____

_____

_____

_____

_____

_____

_____

_____

_____

_____

_____

_____

_____

_____

_____

_____

_____

_____

_____

Day Five

"Trust in the Lord with all thine heart; and lean not on your own understanding. In all thy ways acknowledge him, and he shall direct thy paths." (Proverbs 3:5-6 KJV)

That certainly sounds easy enough. Trusting with ALL your heart is a little different. It really is back to that committing, praying and trusting thing for me. Right about now I want to say, "Thanks God, I'll take it from here."

A few places in the word he mentions not to think more of yourself than we ought to. It also says to love our neighbor as we love ourselves. He must have known healthy opinions of yourself would be difficult. I know *"as a man thinketh in his heart, so is he."* (Proverbs 23:7 KJV) I must learn to "thinketh" differently. I write in my first book about having trouble even remembering my affirmations long enough to say them. It is imperative I learn to see myself as God sees me. But even this I cannot do without him.

The diet I am presently on is very low calories with weighed and measured food. So I am responsible for some part of this diet journey; but, I am trying to think of myself like my Daddy does and look to him for the rest. I have just completed two days of the diet and I have lost 8 pounds. I better not lean on my own understanding now, because that would make no sense.

"Dear Daddy, thank you for my weight loss; but, mostly thank you that I don't have to do this alone. You actually want me to lean on you. That kind of sounds opposite than what the world teaches. Thank you that I can trust you to direct my path this day."

What will you struggle with today?

_____

_____

_____

_____

_____

_____

_____

_____

_____

_____

_____

_____

_____

_____

_____

_____

_____

_____

_____

_____

_____

Day Six

"His mercy is new every morning." (Lamentations 3:22-24)

I t is so funny, but, if I don't say that out loud every morning, someone will say it to me. I think God really wants me to hear that. The actual words are talking about his great faithfulness to us. A few of the interpretations speak to us about not being "consumed". I spent many, many years being consumed by my weight.

A few years ago I printed out some forty-years-ago old photos of myself. They had remained on a composite sheet but were never printed because I thought they made me look too fat. When I look at that pretty young lady in a bathing suit it almost makes me cry. So much of my life was wasted on negative thoughts that were just not true. Negative and false are bad adjectives for such a wonderful life.

Then I tried to fix it. I would diet, exercise, "visualize" and basically try everything I knew to change. It never dawned on me to look to God. That sounds so bad to me now; but, I really thought he had better things to do than listen to me cry over my weight. After all, he must have known it was all my fault.

So my awareness of his mercy towards me is something new. Mercy I don't deserve. Mercy I take for granted most days. But it's new every day. Today I am going to be consumed with remembering his mercy.

"Dear Daddy, thank you that I am learning how much you love me. Thank you for your mercy that is new every single day. I need that mercy for so many details in my life, probably more often than hourly, but most of all now during my quick diet. Please remind me today that you are in control and what you ask of me is to ask you. Please bless all who read this today. Help them remember your mercy towards them."

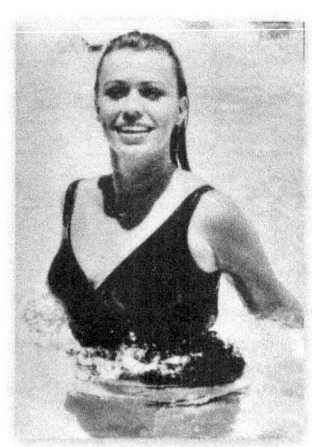

Who will you look to today for mercy? Want to talk it out with God?

_____

_____

_____

_____

_____

_____

_____

_____

_____

_____

_____

_____

_____

_____

_____

_____

_____

_____

_____

_____

_____

_____

_____

Day Seven

"It is the Lord who goes before you. He will be with you: he will not leave or forsake you. Do not fear or be dismayed" (Deuteronomy 31:8 ESV)

Atlanta is my home, so it sure seemed to me that the Lord had a real sense of humor when he had me open a small health food store way down deep in southern Georgia, just about the time I thought I was going to retire. We do really only see parts of our life at a time. Maybe that too is a blessing.

When I signed the long-term lease on the larger space in the shopping center, I couldn't get out of bed. My precious missionary husband, David, asked if God had told me to rent that second space. When I answered that I *thought* so, he said I should spend some time with him to *know* so. I was sitting up reading in the bed, ok, not exactly reading, more like flipping the pages muttering against my husband's boldness to tell ME to seek God. When I looked down at the page of the <u>Bible</u>, there was that word. It would be more appropriate to say, "There was his Word for me."

It is rather early in this round of my diet journey to be pulling this scripture out, but it is like his mercy being new every day. I need a lot of help. Today is day five of the Very Low Calorie Diet and I have lost 10 pounds. So that means I lost 10 pounds in four days of dieting. That really is phenomenal; so why, pray tell, did I fight being disappointed at only ½ pound weight loss this morning?

"Dear Father, thank you for the promise to not let go of me, even when I let go of you. You tell me not to fear, but forgive me and "not forsake" me when I do fear. Thank you for such unconditional love."

My biggest personal challenge is to remember to only do my part and let my Daddy do the rest. He said, he would never leave me nor forsake me. Do you think that means you too?

_____

_____

_____

_____

_____

_____

_____

_____

_____

_____

_____

_____

_____

_____

_____

_____

_____

_____

_____

_____

_____

_____

Day Eight

"God is not the author of confusion, but of peace..."
(1 Corinthians 14:33 KJV)

It is actually a little early in my diet to need so desperately to focus on peace. OK, so maybe it is always more important than I realize. I just do so much better in a controlled environment when I am so drastically reducing my calorie intake. Do I sound like I'm whining?

My husband is usually incredibly good about not tempting me with food I cannot have right now while on my diet. It is almost like an alcoholic not making all their friends abstain from drinking in front of them; but, they really would not want to be forced to hang out in a bar. Last night David spontaneously had a guy over to watch football. I do not take it for granted that all that junk food doesn't temp me.

Seriously, I live with a grateful heart about that one. Somewhere along the way I did figure out if you never eat that stuff you will not want it. Then they started eating left-over organic meat and vegetables. Meat and vegetables I love but could not have on my diet. Then I remembered about all we had been talking about leaning on

God instead of me, trusting in him instead of my will power, and being grateful for his mercy that is new just for today.

Peace was what I needed and peace is what I sought and received. After five days of actual dieting, I have lost 12 pounds!

Thank you that you will never leave me nor forsake me, even when I whine.

_____

_____

_____

_____

_____

_____

_____

_____

_____

_____

_____

_____

_____

_____

_____

_____

_____

_____

_____

_____

_____

_____

Day Nine

"So if you think you are standing firm, be careful that you don't fall. No temptation has overtaken you except what is common to mankind. And God is faithful; he will not let you be tempted beyond what you can bear. But when you are tempted, he will also provide a way out so that you can endure it." (1 Corinthians 10:12-13 NIV)

I write these scary words this morning because it is my nature to take back control. 12 ½ pounds weight loss in less than a week is better than I have ever done. But right here is where I could get in trouble if I am not careful. This week I have done everything I was supposed to, but nothing different than all the other 21 day rounds of this diet. After gratefully maintaining 100 pounds weight loss now going into my fourth year, I know how to do this diet. It would be easy to think this success was something I was doing right. But why better this week than the other 21 day rounds I have done in the past?

What is different? My only explanation is that I am praying more for the words to share with you. In doing so, I am reminding myself that I cannot do this diet on my own and I certainly cannot share with you what I don't have. What I do have is a grateful heart this morning and I feel a warning to keep a humble spirit.

"Dear Lord...there it is. I want you to be Lord of my life today. Not just my diet, but my attitude. Please forgive me for pride."

Day Nine

Please write out your temptations and how you plan to handle them. His mercy is new every day. Thank you, God.

_____

_____

_____

_____

_____

_____

_____

_____

_____

_____

_____

_____

_____

_____

_____

_____

_____

_____

_____

_____

_____

_____

_____

Day Ten

"Thus saith the Lord God; Repent, and turn yourselves from your idols; and turn away your faces from all your abominations." (Ezekiel 14:6 KJV)

According to Wikipedia the word repent combines the two meanings of time and change, after and different, to mean 'to think differently after'. To repent actually means to change ones mind differently from the former thought; a change of mind accompanied by regret and change of conduct, "change of mind and heart", or "change of consciousness".

This morning I woke early worrying about my weight loss. Since I started writing each day AS I AM DIETING, it really is forcing me to be very transparent. What if I gain weight one day? Will I share that in print? It happens, you know, just for no apparent reason. Today I woke early to fret about that. Then I remembered, wasn't I going to "thinketh" differently this time?

If I believe God's word then I should act in a different way to get different results. So before I got out of bed, I quit reasoning about my diet. It is my responsibility to prepare and comply with the rules. Then

I should repent from stressing out over the part I have absolutely no control over. The only thing different about this round of my dieting is that thought. I need to do my part and leave the results to my loving Father.

So I repented. I repented for one more time starting to take back control of something I know very well I cannot fix. I have been on a diet since third grade and I cannot do this. What were their idols in Biblical times? What makes me think it is OK with the Lord if I focus on my weight loss? So I repented for all my fretting. Then I weighed. I have lost 14.6 pounds in one week. How totally crazy is that?

"Dear Father, please forgive me for taking back control of my weight, my diet and this book. You have such a wonderful plan for me and I want to trust only you. I realize it makes you sad when I focus on anything more than your love for me, and the way you provide for all of my needs. This morning I am asking you to forgive me for my lack of trust and I am turning away from any thought that I need to control the outcome of my obedience. From this day forward I am going to ask you to meet all my needs. Show me the next right thing to do this day. Thank you for my astonishing weight loss this past week. You are a good Daddy and I have such a grateful heart."

What are your idols?

_____

_____

_____

_____

_____

_____

_____

_____

_____

_____

_____

_____

_____

_____

_____

_____

_____

_____

_____

_____

_____

_____

_____

_____

Day Eleven

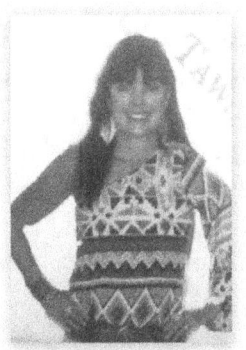

"For the thing which I greatly feared is come upon me, and that which I was afraid of is come unto me." (Job 3:25 KJV)

My close girlfriend, Sissy, can make me laugh so quickly and David often says I should just hire her for entertainment. She lost her father a few years ago, much earlier than expected. This event greatly influenced my intentional time with my Mother every other day. Sissy just kept sobbing that losing her Daddy was her biggest daily fear. I recall thinking of this scripture. Certainly there is no judgment here, for I work at holding my thoughts captive every single day. It is not easy to think about what you are thinking about.

Life gets in the way for me. Yesterday I worked too late and then ate too late, and too little. This morning I am hungry and tired and have gained .2 of a pound. OK, I know how that sounds. It is less than ½ pound, but I GAINED weight for all I did right yesterday. This scripture came to mind. Pastor Henry Wright, author of <u>Be In Health,</u> was the first to make me question what it is that I fear most. It was a few years ago when I realized my greatest fear was to gain more weight.

One would think my greatest fear would be the loss of David or my only son, my daughter-in-love or even my precious granddaughter. Maybe it even should be. It would also make more sense for my greatest fear to be a dreaded disease, or maybe even the state of the affairs in this crazy world. But, weight gain as your greatest fear? Now that just is not right.

If the whole "as a man thinketh in his heart" part is true, then this must be also. I am going to make a better effort at thinking things that are truth. Truth is God loves me and only has my very best in mind. He is always right here with me and in me and I can lean on him all day. He may allow things to attempt to trip me, but he promises to even use all that for my good. So today I will remember I have lost over 14 pounds in one week. That really is astounding. Fear has no place in my diet or anywhere in my life. I am a precious child of The King and today I will meditate on that.

"Father, please forgive me for thinking at all about my weight loss today. I repent for the fear I had yesterday and thank you that your mercy is new every day. You have told me you will stay right here with me so I will not try to figure out anything except your perfect will for me today. I surrender, again, the outcome of my diet and thank you that you are in control and not me. Thank you for loving me so much."

What are your greatest fears?

Day Twelve

"Ask and it will be given to you; seek and you will find; knock and the door will be opened to you. For everyone who asks receives; the one who seeks finds; and to the one who knocks, the door will be opened." (Mathew 7:7-8 (NKJV)

So there it is again. It seems God does not want me to figure it all out. That thought alone goes against my personality. Doesn't society encourage that? He often speaks of being like a little child. If God made me, then he already knows all of my thoughts. Why then should I have to seek him, or ask him? Maybe it is a humbling process. Maybe it is obedience. What I do know is God cannot lie.

A few years ago I was scheduled to speak to a ladies conference about two hours outside of Atlanta in a southern country retreat in the woods. David and I were newly married and living in his southern Alabama. I used this speaking engagement as an opportunity to come back to the city early and spend a few days with Della, my precious prayer partner of many years.

When it was time to leave Della, I was in eight lanes of traffic going over seventy miles an hour when I realized my directions were in my suitcase, in the trunk. I was whimpering out loud when I heard God say, "Let me do it for you." I had recently read someone else say he said that to them once. Then all of a sudden I started saying those words over and over, only each time emphasizing a different word.

"Let *me* do it for you. Let me *do* it for you. Let me do *it* for you. Let me do it *for* you. Let me do it for *you!*"

OK God, you do it. It made me laugh out loud.

In speeding traffic I looked in the lane next to me just as a large bus passed with the name of the church I was to speak for at their ladies retreat. One lady locked eyes with me out the window of the church bus. That lady was the pastor's wife. I followed the bus for two hours out of the city and into the woods. What a good God we serve.

So today, I will seek to do his perfect will and to just BE in his loving arms. I will ask him for everything I need and knock expecting him to open all doors he wants opened to me this day.

"Dear Daddy, thank you that your mercy is new every single day. Please forgive me for trying to take back control, and help me as I seek your perfect will in my life, just for today. I am asking for more weight loss and have a very grateful heart for the 15 pounds so far. I am your temple and I want to be strong and healthy for you. Ok, maybe also for me. Thank you for your great love for me and I am expecting to receive good today."

Will you join me as I expect to receive?

_____

_____

_____

_____

_____

_____

_____

_____

_____

_____

_____

_____

_____

_____

_____

_____

_____

_____

_____

_____

_____

Day Thirteen

"For the Spirit God gave us does not make us timid, but gives us power, love and self-discipline." (2 Timothy 1:7 NIV)

Today I am stalled on my diet. I have neither lost weight nor have I gained. Right here is where I have a choice. In past rounds, I have silently gone into despair. Haven't I done everything correctly? Haven't I made all the right food choices in the right categories? Didn't I even decline the allowed fruit yesterday? Blah, blah, blah...

I bet God gets tired of hearing me whine.

"Thank you Lord that your mercy is new everyday and I can count on today's mercy. I commit to think on that. Thank you I am not in charge, but rather you are. I love the way your son, King David, would carry on about all his woes and dramatically lament over his bed being covered in tears. Then he would say, 'but my God!' and remember all you have done specifically for him in the past. Thank you for my *incredible* weight loss. Thank you for all the blessings that go with that weight loss. Thank you for your spirit of self-discipline. Thank you that I know I am not alone on this diet, but my God!"

Where will your power come from today?

_____

_____

_____

_____

_____

_____

_____

_____

_____

_____

_____

_____

_____

_____

_____

_____

_____

_____

_____

Day Fourteen

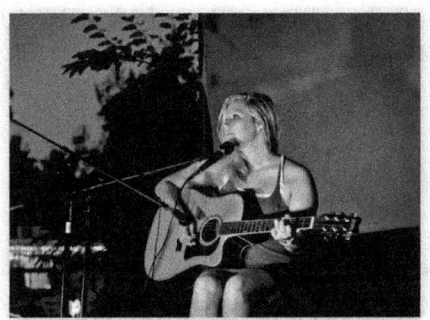

"Speaking to yourselves in psalms and hymns and spiritual songs, singing and making melody in your heart to the Lord. Giving thanks always for all things unto God and the Father in the name of our Lord Jesus Christ; submitting yourselves one to another in the fear of God" (Ephesians 5:19-21 KJV)

That scripture just kept on going. I woke this morning thinking of the first verse; but, when I was looking it up to quote it correctly I just kept typing. The part running around in my head was about the singing and making melody in your heart to the Lord. I was pondering on how difficult it is for me to sing when I am upset.

Do you still remember theme songs from your childhood? I can still sing the Andy Griffith Show, Gilligan's Island, and even The Brady

Bunch. There appears to be a memory component to your brain that remembers catchy tunes better than facts. There are many stories of people with Alzheimer's unable to remember their family members, but can sing every word of the hymn Amazing Grace.

My precious singer/songwriter "almost daughter" of mine, Hananel, recorded herself singing the fruits of the Spirit so I could memorize them. She sang in her crystal clear angelic voice, "Love, joy, peace, patience, kindness, goodness, faithfulness, gentleness and self control." It was amazing how simple it made it for me to remember something I had secretly struggled with for many years.

So what about the bad songs? Do we remember them too? David and I laugh about some of the words of the songs of our youth like "I'm a loser". Is there any wonder many of my generation had such a hard time with life? If there is any truth in the law of attraction and the biblical truth of "as a man thinketh in his heart, so is he", then isn't the negative flipside also truth?

So today I want to sing a song of praise to the Lord, and to you. This is a new day and I am excited about your life and mine. God has a good plan and I want to sing about it with joy and thanksgiving. We are to speak to each other in songs and hymns and spiritual songs. But notice we are to give thanks always to the Lord.

"Dear Father, thank you for the gift of song. Thank you that it ministers to our hearts in a way you understand. Please help me today to only speak in encouraging ways to others, and to myself. Thank you that your mercy is new just for today and that I can choose to rest in it. Thank you for my weight loss of 17 more pounds and the truth that you care about what matters to me. Please help me this day to care more about what matters to you."

Do you have a song for today?

_____

_____

_____

_____

_____

_____

_____

_____

_____

_____

_____

_____

_____

_____

_____

_____

_____

_____

_____

_____

Day Fifteen

"Rejoice in the Lord always. Again I say, rejoice! Let your gentleness be known to all men. The Lord is at hand. Be anxious for nothing, but in everything by prayer and supplication, with thanksgiving, let your requests be known to God; and the peace of God, which surpasses all understanding, will guard your hearts and minds through Christ Jesus." (Philippians 4:4 NKJV)

Before David and I married and moved to Alabama and before we were so blessed to move to this beautiful sanctuary in South Georgia, Atlanta was my home. I grew up in that fabulous city. My friend, Mark, was the first person I ever saw actually carry his <u>Bible</u> with him. He owned a radio station in the city and said if he didn't take his <u>Bible</u> with him (and it was a big one!) he would forget. I asked what it was he would forget. He explained he would take back control of his life just as soon as God started moving.

"Thanks God, I'll take it from here."

That's me. It's not my intent, but it does seem to be my nature. I have not been on my actual low calorie diet but for two weeks; yet, I have stalled twice now. Again I did not gain (yay!) but also I did not lose any weight yesterday. Everything was done exactly by the rules, yet I did not get what I wanted. The fact I have lost 17 pounds in less than two weeks is not enough for me. Do you see how psycho that sounds?

So today I will make a conscience effort to rejoice in the Lord, remind him what I really want and expect his peace to guard my heart. My Daddy really loves me.

"Dear Father, thank you that you are right here. Thank you that I do not have to go anywhere to find you, or go through anyone to talk with you. Thank you that you love me so much that sometimes you don't give me what I want just when I want it. Forgive me for not trusting your timing more. Today I ask for your peace; the kind that comes from your mercy that is new every day. Please help me be obedient to my part in this diet, and give you back all the rest of it. Thank you for my incredible weight loss and I ask for more when it is in your perfect will. Thank you, Lord, that you love me."

What do you want today? Tell Daddy.

_____

_____

_____

_____

_____

_____

_____

_____

_____

_____

_____

_____

_____

_____

_____

_____

_____

_____

_____

_____

Day Sixteen

"Finally, brethren, whatever things are true, whatever things are noble, whatever things are just, whatever things are pure, whatever things are lovely, whatever things are of good report, if there is any virtue and if there is anything praiseworthy – meditate on these things." (Philippians 4:8)

As the owner of a small health food store in South Georgia during an economic recession, I know firsthand how difficult it can be to not worry. It almost seems like we are supposed to worry. I see many people in my private practice who have been trained to worry; even young Mothers who overmedicate their children just as a precaution. I'm not sure where we came up with this idea, but I know it was not God's.

This crazy diet I am back on for three weeks (see <u>30 Pounds in 3 Weeks...and the Diets I Use to Maintain 100 Pound Weight Loss</u>) requires that you do not exercise for the three weeks during the "very low calorie" part. After stalling my loss a few times over something silly like a good song turning my walking in the swimming pool into dancing, I now take even that part seriously. It seems like ALL the rules are serious for serious weight loss. Yesterday I walked too much.

So if I believe any of the <u>Bible</u>, I must believe all of it. We have been told so many times not to worry about anything. We have now been told not to even think about things negative. God instructs us to meditate on and fill our minds with things true, noble, reputable, authentic, compelling, gracious – the best, not the ugly; things to praise, not things to curse. I had trouble sleeping last night thinking about the staff schedule and about excessive walking. Before I even got on the scales this morning, I finally made a decision to do all these things.

This is a good diet and I have been very successful on it for years now. I am going to expect the best. My health food store has never been mine, but just obedience to what the Lord told me to do. I am going to expect the best there too.

I weighed and am down another pound. Let's meditate on his goodness, even when I forget.

"Dear Daddy, thank you that you are so merciful to me again today. Forgive me when I try to take back control and only remember my mistakes. Thank you for my weight loss and how you have helped me through these last few days. Thank you that I don't have to do anything on my own."

Will you think about what you are thinking about today? Maybe it would help to write it out.

_____

_____

_____

_____

_____

_____

_____

_____

_____

_____

_____

_____

_____

_____

_____

_____

_____

_____

_____

_____

Day Seventeen

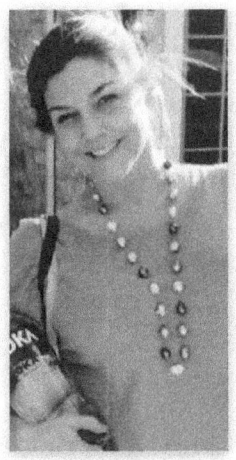

"If ye then be risen with Christ, seek those things which are above, where Christ sitteth on the right hand of God. Set your affection on things above, not on things on the earth." (Colossians 3:1-2 KJV)

S ometimes that is hard for me. Ok, usually that is hard for me. There are so many things going on in my life at one time, often I get distracted. My very profound friend Ellen, in Dallas, feels distractions are one of our biggest enemies. I am not sure I ever thought about it exactly that way but, I believe she is completely correct. Since attempting to write these few words, I have had three texts and four phone calls. Every one of them are important; but, distractions compete for my attention. These are times I think of Ellen and pray for her.

Today, I really want to keep my mind and my affection towards things of God and not this world. I once heard the urgent will win out over the important if I do not make a conscience effort. It all seems important to me. There is no way I can discern the difference on my own. It surely is a good, great, God thing that I am not alone.

This is the end of two weeks on my diet and I have lost 19.5 pounds. There is no way I could have done that!

Wow, it seems this prayer stuff really does work.

"Dear Father, thank you that your mercy is new just for today. Thank you that you will help me keep my mind on you. I need help in holding back the distractions of this world. My desire is to focus on you and your perfect will, just for today. Thank you for my incredible weight loss and it makes me cry thinking about how much you love me. Please help me show others today how much you love them."

What will you think about today?

_____

_____

_____

_____

_____

_____

_____

_____

_____

_____

_____

_____

_____

_____

_____

_____

_____

_____

_____

_____

_____

_____

Day Eighteen

"And whatever you do in word or deed, do all in the name of the Lord Jesus, giving thanks to God the Father through Him." (Colossians 3:17 NKJV)

The Message Bible says, "Let every detail in your lives – words, actions, whatever – be done in the name of the Master, Jesus, thanking God the Father every step of the way." Maybe the "whatever" even means thoughts? How can such simple words be so hard? I gained a pound.

Remember in the beginning of this diet journey, I said my part was just to keep the rules and look to God for the rest? Well, it gets tough when you gain and not lose. Ok, it is just a pound and I know all the variables that could be involved in just a pound of weight gain. I woke up this morning promising to trust God in whatever. So I choose to thank him.

I thank him for my success on this incredible diet. I thank him for my good health. I thank him for never leaving me nor forsaking me. I thank him that I am not alone. I thank him for the comfort of his words to me.

I thank him for the freedom to talk about his goodness. I thank him for the written Word.

"Dear Father, thank you that I do not have to figure out life without you. Thank you for my weight loss on this diet. You know I am not happy about gaining a pound yesterday, but you also know I am really trying to trust you in this. I do know you have my best interest in mind and that you will make it all good for me. Thank you that you will not leave me alone and that your mercy is new just for today. I choose to be excited about what you are doing in my life. "

What are you thankful for today?

_____

_____

_____

_____

_____

_____

_____

_____

_____

_____

_____

_____

_____

_____

_____

_____

_____

_____

_____

_____

_____

Day Nineteen

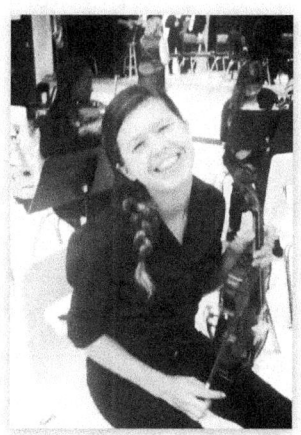

"I thank my God every time I remember you. In all my prayers for all of you, I always pray with joy because of your partner-ship in the gospel from the first day until now, being confident of this, that he who began a good work in you will carry it on to completion until the day of Christ Jesus." (Philippians 1:3-6 NIV)

I t is often in my life that I remind God of that last part. In crying out to him for my son, my niece and now my granddaughter, Helena, I remind God frequently that he started it and he promised to complete it. Every day I pray he will be real in their lives. I do pray this with confidence because the Lord cannot lie.

Since starting this diet this round, while writing to you, I have reminded him again for you and me. I am his, the results of this diet are all his business and I am confident that he who began a good thing will complete it. See how important it is to speak his Word. I lost the 1 pound yesterday, and then one more. I expect him to take care of me.

"Dear Daddy, thank you that you make yourself real in my life. Even when I wandered off, you came after me. Please be real to my loved ones and to all who read these words. Thank you for your mercy that is new every day. Thank you for this diet, and the way you never leave me to do it alone. Help me to remember today how much you love me and to expect only the best in my world and in those who matter to me. Please help everyone matter to me."

What do you expect today?

_____
_____
_____
_____
_____
_____
_____
_____
_____
_____
_____
_____
_____
_____
_____
_____
_____
_____
_____

Day Twenty

"Have no fear of sudden disaster or of the ruin that overtakes the wicked, for the Lord will be at your side and will keep your foot from being snared." (Proverbs 3:25-26 NIV)

Remembering theses words are extra important to me at this stage in my diet. Ok, it is important all of the time to remember that the Lord is always at my side; but, when I get on the home stretch of this three and a half week diet, I can get anxious if I am not con-science of my thoughts. What if I don't lose any more weight this last week? What if I gain? What if I let everyone down with my numbers?

So I did only lose ½ of a pound yesterday, but that is still losing. I seem to always come back to the same thoughts: I cannot do this on my own and no matter how hard I try, I cannot influence the weight loss on this particular diet. My part seems to be to follow the rules and leave the results to my Daddy who is going to "keep my foot from being snared."

Did you ever notice how many times we were told not to fear? Fear appears to be at the root of most disease. The first time I read that, I stopped and pondered what I was really afraid of. I raised my son as a single Mom, so I have known a special kind of fear; fear of the unknown for our safety and well being. You would think I would now fear the loss of my precious husband or my granddaughter, Helena, or maybe even my business I have worked so hard to create and build. In my private practice I see wonderful people with terrible diseases almost every day. But when I really tried to identify what my most prevalent personal fear was, I realized it was fear of gaining more weight. How crazy is that? Of all the acceptable woes to stress over, my main fear is weight gain. I really had to take a long hard look at that one.

Either everything God said is true or none of it is. There are over 365 "fear nots" in the <u>Bible</u>, and that is not even counting all the times we were told not to be anxious and not to worry. I was almost forty years old when I heard for the first time that there was nothing I could do to make God love me more. The flip side of that is true also. There is nothing I can do to make him love me less. Any parent knows that one. We may be disappointed in something our child is doing, but we don't love them any less.

So if God's love for me is free for the accepting, wouldn't I be rather foolish to live in fear of not having it? It is rather sad that I am just now pulling all these pieces together about how his unfailing love relates to my weight. Maybe I thought God had better things to do then to listen to me whine about weight. Maybe I could listen to him more and whine less. Ouch!

"Dear Daddy, thank you that you love me no matter what I weigh. Thank you that you are not even upset with me for the struggles I have understanding how much you love me. Forgive me for not trusting you more. Today I am going to practice the part about not fearing anyone or anything. Thank you for my continued weight loss."

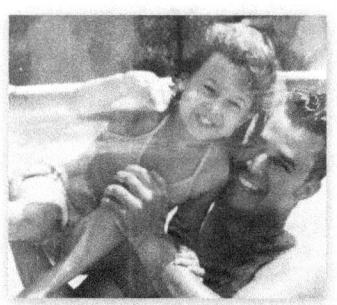

Can you identify your fears? Maybe you could write them down and give them all to your Daddy.

_____

_____

_____

_____

_____

_____

_____

_____

_____

_____

_____

_____

_____

_____

_____

_____

_____

_____

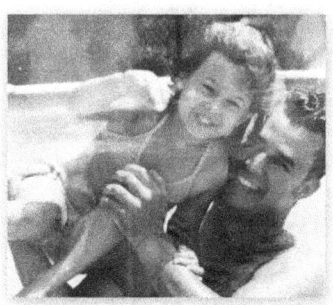

Can you identify your fears? Maybe you could write them down and give them all to your Daddy.

_____

_____

_____

_____

_____

_____

_____

_____

_____

_____

_____

_____

_____

_____

_____

_____

_____

_____

Day Twenty-One

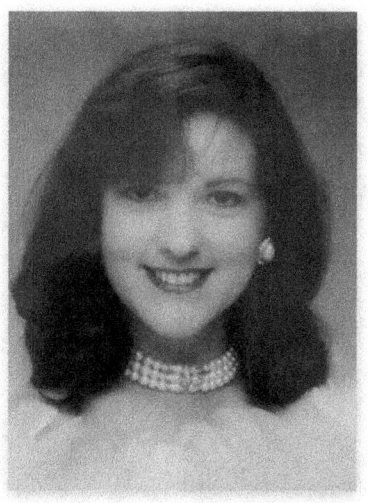

"Blessed shall you be when you come in, and blessed shall you be when you go out." (Deuteronomy 28:6 NKJV)

Those were the words Della prayed over me the first time I went to her house to meet her and some of her girlfriends. They met every week to pray for their children, their children's teachers, the schools and the school system in the city of Atlanta. It was a powerful time around Della's little kitchen table.

These ladies taught me how to pray. I remember in detail how awkward I felt when I first arrived in my business suit to pray with perfect strangers. My eyes popped open when the quiet young mother in the cotton dress thanked God for the little yellow flower he left her by the sidewalk that morning. Most of their prayers were just like that. Simple and honest were the prayers to a real Father from the desperate Moms who really were in touch with their Daddy. They prayed their hearts with expectations.

They expected God to be good to his word. They expected God to answer every honest prayer. They expected God to not show favoritism or disinterest with any of their prayers. They got results too!

Of course I had to leave early and go to work, and that is when Della prayed those words over me. "Lord please bless her going out and her coming in." I knew she was someone I wanted to be praying for me. It has been many, many years now and Della and I still pray together. But what she taught me was the power of praying God's words. When I found those words in scripture, it made me cry. Della always prays scripture over me.

"Father, thank you for your Word. Thank you that you care about everything in my life. Thank you for your gentle nudging to go where you want me to go and to be obedient to your desires for my life. Thank you for your mercy towards me, especially when I don't get it all right. Thank you that you love me so much. I really want to know you better, to love you more. Thank you for another pound of weight loss."

God wants to bless me. He wants to bless you. So…I pray that our Daddy bless your going out and your coming in. May everything you desire today line up perfectly with his will for your life.

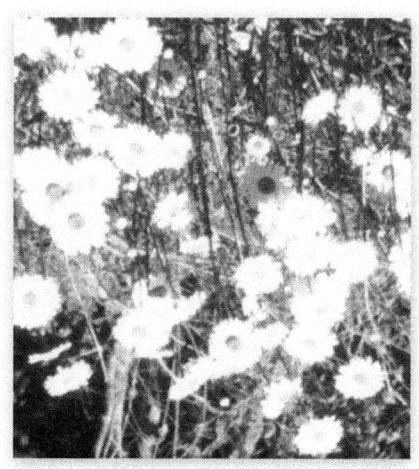

What is your prayer for today?

_____

_____

_____

_____

_____

_____

_____

_____

_____

_____

_____

_____

_____

Day Twenty-Two

"The Spirit of the Lord is upon me, because he has anointed me to preach the gospel to the poor; he has sent me to heal the brokenhearted, to proclaim liberty to the captives and recovery of sight to the blind, to set at liberty those who are oppressed; to proclaim the acceptable year of the Lord...Today this Scripture is fulfilled in your hearing." (Luke 4: 18-21 NKJV)

I take most of the <u>Bible</u> literally. I say most not because I don't believe every single word, it just seems to me there are some true things written that were not meant literally. But these scriptures are not part of that to me. Jesus said these words and he is the Word. He was talking about himself and he was talking to me.

He has called me to speak truth about his Word. That he is truth and he cannot lie. I have been the poor; both in possessions and in spirit. When my teenage husband left me with a sick baby and I lay crouched in fear on the floor sobbing for days, I was poor and brokenhearted. God himself was right there with me.

For over fifty years I was blind to my obsession with my weight. The pictures I see of myself as a young woman almost make me cry. I was so perfect. My negative thoughts about my body held me captive, they consumed my every thought. His words were always there for me. I just forgot. I was a captive to a deceiver. It never crossed my mind to wonder what the Lord said about me.

He said I was made in his image. Do I think he is fat? He "knew me before he made me". Would he have made me anything but pleasing to him? I am the "apple of his eye" and that really doesn't sound like I should be lacking in anything. He wants me to "prosper and be in good health", and I know he cannot lie. So maybe those words of Jesus so many years ago are still completely true today. These scriptures are being fulfilled today in the person of Jesus. Today is the acceptable year of the Lord.

"Dear Father, please forgive me for my doubts. Please forgive all the times I only believed part of what you said. Thank you for your mercy towards me; in all my failings to be all you have in your heart for me. Thank you that your mercy is fresh and new every morning. Please help me to see me the way you do. Thank you for my success on my diet. Thank you that you are setting my heart free."

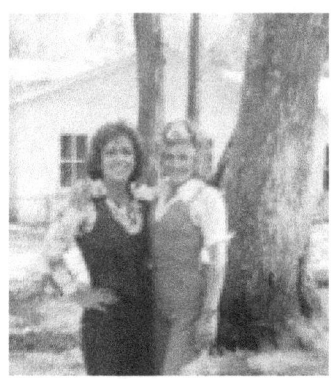

Do you see a fat person? Do you believe God; everything he says?

_____

_____

_____

_____

_____

_____

_____

_____

_____

_____

_____

_____

_____

_____

_____

_____

_____

Day Twenty-Three

"A man's stomach shall be satisfied from the fruit of his mouth; from the produce of his lips he shall be filled. Death and life are in the power of the tongue, and those who love it will eat its fruit." (Proverbs 18:20-21 NKJV)

David and I were reading Song of Solomon this morning and I told him to never compare MY hair to a herd of goats. We had a good laugh about those words in the <u>Bible</u>. They were obviously written when that was a compliment. I wonder how often we say things without thinking about the whole "power of life and death in the tongue" thing. I know I have really been guilty of this in the past.

Our music of the sixties and seventies had a huge impact on society. We had some truly great musicians of all time, but we did chant some pretty dark stuff. What about this one: "I'm a loser...I'm not what I appear to be." Excuse me, but there is no wonder we had so much trouble just growing up.

One of my recent clients with stage four rectal cancer shared with me how every day of her marriage she voiced what a pain in her butt his family was to her. Unfortunately I frequently hear beautiful women "hating their breasts" only to have those same breasts lost to breast cancer. I want to learn this one easier.

A young lady I barely knew said that she bet my Mother told me I was beautiful. She did and she does. Mother has always said you tell a child who they will be. She has no tolerance for parents professing negatives to their children. I told my son every day of his life in my home how much his absent father loved him.

How about these: God holds me in his hands so I am not afraid. He wants me to prosper and be in good health. I am the righteousness of Christ. I do not get discouraged because God is with me wherever I go. I am in right standing with God because of Christ. I am happy as I walk in the light of God's presence. As I cling to God in confidence, I receive his mercy and grace. In the morning I share my requests with God and wait in eager expectation for what he will do. In my soul and spirit I am being renewed day by day.

"Dear Father, please help my friends know who they are. Thank you for loving me and helping me with my diet. Please help me finish well."

How do you bless you?

_____

_____

_____

_____

_____

_____

_____

_____

_____

_____

_____

_____

_____

_____

_____

_____

_____

_____

_____

_____

_____

_____

Day Twenty-Four

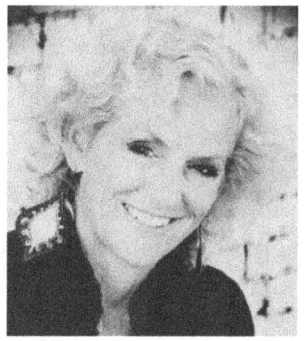

"It is written: "I believed; therefore I have spoken." Since we have that same spirit of faith, we also believe and therefore speak." (2 Corinthians 4:13 NIV)

t is so very important to watch how we speak. One of my closest friends for many years, Robin, wrote a book recently on <u>The Believer's Guide to the Law of Attraction.</u> She really does a thorough job in explaining this principle. Sometimes it is easier for me to believe the theory than to put these truths into action. First thing in the morning I set my mind to be joyful and kind and speak only affirming words to others. Then I have to get out of bed.

The truths are all there in Scripture. The truth about who Jesus is and what he did for me is all written in that same chapter. *"All this is for your benefit, so that the grace that is reaching more and more people may cause thanksgiving to overflow to the glory of God. Therefore we do not lose heart..."*

The "economic downturn" really hit us hard in South Georgia. Remember that I have my private practice in my little health food store. A retail store in a small town deep in the South is not exactly where I would choose to be in an economic recession. I had just spent a few years in counseling to try to learn how not to be a workaholic. Then I married, moved to this precious small town and opened a health food store. Then the recession affected everyone. God has a real sense of humor.

Yesterday, I had two extremely difficult business traumas. This morning I have gained a little over ½ pound; and all that business stress from the past few years is coming to a head this day. Oh yeah, I also have private consultations with wonderful clients every half hour all day and well into the night. I have some choices right here. Either everything he said is true or none of it is.

Further down in that same chapter he writes, *"Therefore we do not lose heart, even though our outward man is perishing, yet the inward man is being renewed day by day. For our light affliction, which is but for a moment, is working for us a far more exceeding and eternal weight of glory, while we do not look at the things which are seen, but at the things which are not seen. For the things which are seen are temporary, but the things which are not seen are eternal."* (NKJV)

"Dear Daddy, I know I can do very little of any of this myself. For years I tried everything my way and it did not make me happy. I want the peace you promise from looking to you. Forgive me for even trying to figure it all out. I know you love me and I am excited about what you are doing in my life. Today I will speak of your greatness."

How can we make those ideals reality in our life today?

_____

_____

_____

_____

_____

_____

_____

_____

_____

_____

_____

_____

_____

_____

_____

_____

_____

_____

_____

_____

_____

Day Twenty-five

"...You do not have because you do not ask God. When you do not receive, because you ask with wrong motives that you may spend what you get on your pleasures." (James 2-3 NIV)

Ok, I am not going to pretend for a moment that I do not want to lose weight for my pleasure. Really nothing taste as good as thin feels; not that I have ever known what "thin" actually is. Something happened in my heart a few years ago and I now have a new motive for weight loss other than just vanity. I really am the temple of the living God and I need my body to be strong and healthy for this thing we call life.

When you are married to a missionary you really do not have a whole lot of options in what you drive. My present SUV is black with dark windows and big wheels. The staff I had at the health food store said something about "pimp my ride." After I lost over 100 pounds, getting in that truck is just no big deal. It was actually after the first 30 pounds that I thought someone had stolen my tires! It really was funny. Climbing into the vehicle was just totally different after my weight loss.

The swimming pool has always been my favorite exercise. My real "aerobic queen" girlfriends could not keep up with some of my moves in the swimming pool. After I lost even some of the weight, I could not stay afloat. I guess I had a good bit of buoyancy before.

So I do not pretend or try to manipulate the Lord about my diet. I want to lose weight for a few really good reasons. I want to look better and feel better in my clothes. I want to travel more (ok, that is already happening) and be more active every day. I want to be a good example of health and a motivator to others. Most of all I want to be all God made me to be.

He loves me the same no matter what size I am. Maybe I am more joyful when there is less of me and more of him.

"Dear Father, thank you that you promised to never leave me nor forsake me. Thank you for being real in my life. Please help all my friends reading these words know how much you love them, just as they are right now. Thank you that you have brand new mercy for me this day, and I ask you to show that mercy also to them today. Thank you I am still losing weight. Please help me this day keep my mind on you."

Why do you want to diet?

_____

_____

_____

_____

_____

_____

_____

_____

_____

_____

_____

_____

_____

_____

_____

_____

_____

_____

_____

_____

Day Twenty-Six

So Jesus answered and said to them, *"Have faith in God. For assuredly, I say to you, whoever says to this mountain, 'Be removed and be cast into the sea,' and does not doubt in his heart, but believes that those things he says will be done, he will have whatever he says. Therefore I say to you, whatever things you ask when you pray, believe that you receive them, and you will have them."* (Mark 11:22-24 NKJV)

Once I saw a cartoon where these little children were holding a family dog saying, "we prayed that he get well, now can we take him out to play." That really has stuck in my memory for years. Why can't I have that simple childlike faith? That is exactly what I want, the kind of faith that moves mountains. The kind of faith that believes my Father in Heaven knows what is best for me.

The end of my diet is coming up tomorrow and I want the kind of faith that I will finish well. I want the kind of faith that if the scales do not say what I want them to say, I will still be happy about my success. My success really is in my attitude now. I love the story of the mustard seed. It is so teeny, yet grows into a huge beautiful plant. I want that.

If I really believe God's word, than I need to ask my Daddy, with confidence and believe that he will give me the desires of my heart when they are what is best for me. When it comes to dieting, I really have to trust the Lord only wants to help me to be all he had in mind when he created me as his own little girl.

After a few years of counseling, my friend asked me why I thought God made me. I answered something about him having something in mind just for me to do with my life. He asked why I had a son. Was it to have someone to take out the trash and help unload the groceries? I said of course not, it was to love. I wanted my son to love. That was the beginning of my trying to understand my God. He just plain loves me. He loves me just like I am and not one bit more when I lose weight.

Every other devotion I have shared with you this month was written first thing each morning. This one is at bedtime. Tonight I am going to sleep consciously asking God to move mountains and believing he only wants good for me. I am excited to see what the scales say in the morning.

"Dear Father, as I get ready to go to sleep tonight, I thank you for the blessings of these past few weeks. Tomorrow is the last day of my diet and I am asking you to let me finish well. In your Bible your new day began at sunset. Thank you for a new beginning and a whole new day of your mercy. Thank you for loving me so much. I want to love you more."

Do you have the faith to move your mountain? Do you believe it only takes the faith of a mustard seed?

_____

_____

_____

_____

_____

_____

_____

_____

_____

_____

_____

_____

_____

_____

_____

_____

_____

_____

_____

Day Twenty-Seven

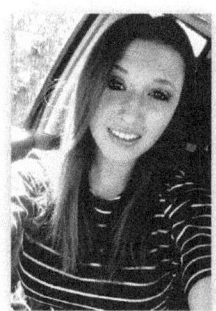

"This Book of the Law shall not depart from your mouth, but you shall meditate in it day and night, that you may observe to do according to all that is written in it. For then you will make your way prosperous, and then you will have good success." (Joshua 1:8 NKJV)

Mine and your salvation is not dependant on anything we can do, but rather on what Jesus has already done for us. When he died on that cross and rose again; he paid the penalty for all my junk. He stood in for me. When my precious niece, Jasmine, was just a very little girl, she asked, "Why DID Jesus die on the cwoss?" (She is grown now and doesn't like me to make fun of her inability to pronounce her "r's" when she was really young.)

She was staring out the car window in deep thought and I answered, "When you do something bad you know someone is going to get in trouble for it." Jesus said, "Do not punish Jasmine, but punish me instead."

Four-year-old Jasmine looked at me with astonishment in those giant dark eyes and exclaimed, "Well, if everyone knew that, everyone would love him!" I never forgot her perfect words. If you want the simple truth, just ask a child.

These promises do seem to be contingent on our doing our part. But maybe our part is not the way others have always condemned us to failure, to "do according to ALL that is written". Maybe the key words really are about meditating on his words day and night and "observing" to do all according to all that is written. That does seem more attainable to me.

If God does really know my heart, and he should, then doesn't he also know my intent? I feel my part is to do the meditating on the truth of the <u>Bible</u> and asking him to do the rest. I accepted the free gift of salvation he offered me when he died on the cross for me. I really want to meditate day and night on all his promises. I really do want my "ways to be prosperous, and have good success."

"Dear Lord, thank you for the free gift you gave me at the cross. Thank you for the way you have so many promises to 'never leave me nor forsake me', even when I mess up. Thank you for your new mercy just for today. Thank you for my incredible weight loss, even if I did gain ½ pound the last day. This 25 and ¾ pound weight loss in only three weeks is impossible on my own. I will meditate on your goodness day and night and expect my way to be prosperous and successful. Please be real to my friends today as they seek to know you better."

I expect God to be true to his Word. What are you expecting today?

_____

_____

_____

_____

_____

_____

_____

_____

_____

_____

_____

_____

_____

_____

_____

_____

_____

_____

_____

_____

Day Twenty-Eight

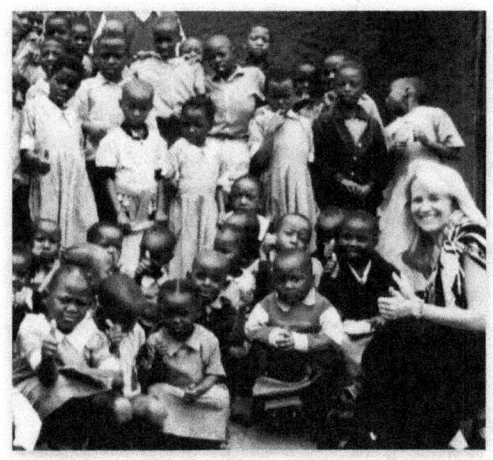

"Now Jabez called on the God of Israel, saying, 'Oh that You would bless me indeed and enlarge my border, and that Your hand might be with me, and that You would keep me from harm that it may not pain me!' And God granted him what he requested." (1 Chronicles 4:10 NASB)

D avid and I were so blessed to have received the little book <u>The Prayer of Jabez</u> from a gorgeous missionary friend from South Africa, Elise, just months after it was released. For over fourteen years we have included that prayer in our daily devotions and have seen miracle after miracle. We were extra blessed to have heard the author, Bruce Wilkinson, himself, teach these obscure scriptures to us.

Those few days were all wonderful and life changing, but the part that impacted me the most was the boldness of the words "bless me"... indeed! Who prays, at least out loud, for God to bless ME? Then the Word says, "and God granted him what he requested." That was so foreign to me. Secretly I wondered how many times I thought myself unworthy of his blessings. So does Jesus have to die again for me to think it is alright for me to claim his blessing? These thoughts were very painful to me.

My little South Georgia health food store is in a popular shopping center. When my staff seats my private clients in my office they call me and I then rush back to my office. Way too many times I am running late and driving too fast into the shopping center and around to the back entrance. Just as I would round the side of the main anchor store I would always pray, "Father, please give me the mind of Christ."

One day I heard God say, "Why do you ask me that every day?" I almost wrecked the truck.

"Well, Lord, because I can do nothing without you; and all things through you." That sounded spiritual enough.

He whispered in my heart, "But why do you ask me for something you already have?" It made me cry.

So I ask myself again, "Does Jesus have to die again for me to think it is alright for me to claim his blessing?"

God granted Jabez what he requested when he asked him to bless him.

"Dear God, please bless me indeed. You know I want to bless others, but you also know I just plain need your help for my life. I cannot live in this world without you every minute of my day. I am asking you to help me make good food choices today. It is like that Centurion saying, 'Lord, I believe; but help me with my unbelief.' Forgive me for thinking there is anything in my life that you are not interested in. I know you love me and I want to love you more."

What about you, can you ask the God of Israel to bless you indeed?

_____

_____

_____

_____

_____

_____

_____

_____

_____

_____

_____

_____

_____

_____

_____

_____

_____

_____

_____

_____

_____

_____

Day Twenty-Nine

"I can do all things through Christ who strengthens me."
(Philippians 4:13 NKJV)

Years ago I resigned a very big job with a Fortune Five-Hundred company. It was after being unemployed for over five months that I took God out of church and really had a heart-to-heart conversation with him. In pretty disrespectful words, I reminded God that I had been talking to him since I was a young girl, yet, he NEVER said anything back to me. I whined on and on and ended my ranting with yelling that I did not need to know the where, when or the how. I just needed him to tell me what he wanted me to do with my blank, blank, blank life. He answered "health food."

It made me so mad. Here I was trying to get God himself to talk with me, and all I could think of was food? Right about then the phone rang in my home in Tampa, Florida where I had been stranded when I quit that big job. It was Bertha of Bertha's Health Foods telling me my special aged garlic formula was back in stock now. She said she was prepared to leave a phone message for me and questioned why I was home in the middle of the week. I explained that I had quit that horrible job and she exclaimed, "Well, praise God, maybe you are supposed to be in the health food industry!"

Are you kidding me? Did she really say "health food"? It was more than I could take in. I started wailing crying as I objected again. It is all pretty entertaining now looking back, but trust me it was not at the time. God really does have such a sense of humor, though probably not the least bit impressed with my tantrum. When the next morning he woke up the man in Houston, Texas and told him to hire Charlene; that almost retired man didn't even know a Charlene. My resume arrived that morning. He flew to Tampa, interviewed me and called from the airport to say he was concerned that I never even asked what this little job paid.

Why did I care what the job paid? It was the very first time I was trying to do things God's way. He said the job covered five states. I muttered something about hoping they were southern states. He then said I would have to move to the city of Atlanta. It made me laugh out-loud as I explained that I grew up in Atlanta, Georgia and my aging grandparents were still there.

Six months later my boss made me speak to all of the sales staff at a meeting in California about how to become number one. I tried my best to avoid actually saying what the real truth was, but ended up just explaining that I had decided to do things God's way, and that I guess he is always number one. A murmur went through the room and I heard, "I think she said God did it!" I cannot understand myself when I forget that truth.

"Thank you, Father, for all your promises for my life. I know you are all my strength and that what you really want from me is to look to you for any and everything. Forgive me for all the times that I act like it's hard to let you do it. Please help me this day to remember to look to you for all my needs. I do not know a lot about submitting to a King; but, I really want to just be your child."

Do you think God cares about your diet?

_____

_____

_____

_____

_____

_____

_____

_____

_____

_____

_____

_____

_____

_____

_____

_____

_____

_____

_____

_____

_____

Day Thirty

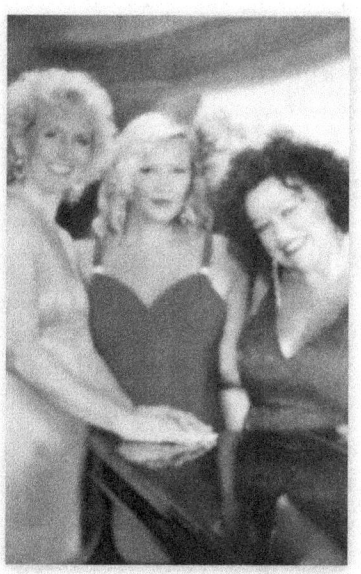

"The steadfast of mind You will keep in perfect peace, because he trusts in You." (Isaiah 26:3 NASB)

I t has been over four years now since I lost that first 100 pounds. Anyone can lose weight and I have done it a "ca-zillion" times; but, this is the first time in my life I have only gained just a little and then gone back on my diet to lose more. I am literally maintaining that 100 pound weight loss for almost five years now.

Not for one moment do I think I am somehow superhuman at this weight loss quest. There are not a lot of rules I follow in my real life; but never, never, never ever do I eat that drug sugar. I do not do heroin or cocaine, and I do not eat sugar.

My sixtieth birthday came around right after I reached that 100 pound weight loss marker. My precious friends Robin and Hananel celebrated with me on a Bahamas cruise. So many were concerned for me since I had just lost the weight. But see, I eat the same no matter where I am. Continuing to drink half my body weight in ounces of water also seems to be crucial to my long term weight loss.

There is no doubt in my mind and heart, and yes, also in my body; this is a God thing. I do believe he cares about my body; after all, he calls it his temple. He holds me in the palm of his hand and even saves every one of my tears. It would be insane to think he doesn't care about my diet. This has cycled right back around to wondering what my part is in this weight loss.

It is my belief that my part is to "cast all my cares on him because he cares for me." It has been argued by many that Jesus did not turn the wine to water; yet, he turned the water to wine. It has also been stated many times in the Bible not to be "drunk" on wine. This is relative to my personal diet in that I cannot eat trigger "foods" (I am not so sure they are real foods.) and not stir up my addiction to the drug sugar. Can you really smoke marijuana and not be "drunk"? Can I really eat sugar and not think about wanting more?

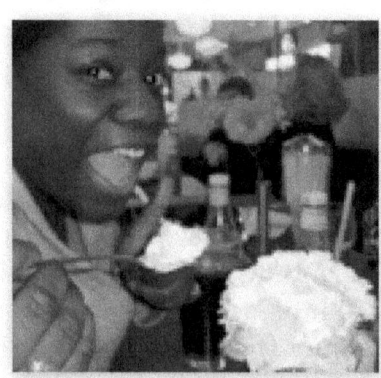

For over thirty years I have been in the natural food industry. I have actually been a Doctor of Natural Health for almost fifteen years now. Over all those years I have always known about sugar, but didn't tell you because I wanted you to like me. This is a true story. Whether the presenting health issue was breast cancer, heart disease, or even dementia I have known for many, many years it could be sugar causing the inflammation response in most disease.

Late at night I would cry out to the Lord about wanting a sweet "Mother Mary" spirit. No one wants to hear a strong Elijah voice talking about everyone giving up their drug of choice. I have gone into this position kicking and screaming.

"Prepare ye the way of the Lord!"

We are his temple. He cares about what matters to us. We are to not be drunk...on anything! (Please love me anyway, but I believe this means sugar too.)

"Father, thank you that you said you would never leave me nor forsake me. Thank you for your new mercy you have set aside for me every day. Forgive me when I try to take back control of EVERYTHING in my life. Please guard my every step as I walk out this total healing you have died for. You know my heart towards all who are reading this. Please, Daddy, bless them with great success."

Your Beautiful Daughter

"For I know the plans I have for you, declares the Lord, plans to prosper you and not to harm you, plans to give you hope and a future. Then you will call on me and come and pray to me, and I will listen to you. You will seek me and find me, when you seek me with all your heart. I will be found by you, declares the Lord..." (Jeremiah 29:11-14 NIV)

_____

_____

_____

_____

_____

_____

_____

_____

_____

_____

_____

_____

_____

_____

_____

_____

_____

_____

_____

_____

_____

_____

_____

_____

_____

_____

_____

_____

_____

_____

_____

_____

_____

_____

_____

_____

_____

_____

_____

_____

_____

_____

_____

www.ingramcontent.com/pod-product-compliance
Lightning Source LLC
Chambersburg PA
CBHW070921290526
45795CB00001B/379